DEDICATION

This book is dedicated to everybody who wants to have stay fit and have a healthy lifestyle.

I also dedicate this book to my loving sister, Angelica. Thank you for inspiring to bring out the best in me.

TABLE OF CONTENTS

Publishers Notes... 2

Dedication 3

Chapter 1- Basic and Essentials of Health.......................... 5

Chapter 2- Your Body and Its Needs 11

Chapter 3- Fitness Armory 20

Chapter 4- Getting Down, Sweaty and Dirty 25

Chapter 5- Machine and Weights Handling......................31

Chapter 6- Novelty Exercise That Do Work 36

Chapter 7- Consistency is the Key 45

Chapter 8- Women and Their Exercise Needs 50

Chapter 9- Now is the Time To Get in Shape!...................55

About The Author..59

Health and Fitness Buff

The Fundamentals on How to Be Fit and Stay Healthy

By: Steve Mallari

9781635013221

PUBLISHERS NOTES

Disclaimer – Speedy Publishing LLC

This publication is intended to provide helpful and informative material. It is not intended to diagnose, treat, cure, or prevent any health problem or condition, nor is intended to replace the advice of a physician. No action should be taken solely on the contents of this book. Always consult your physician or qualified health-care professional on any matters regarding your health and before adopting any suggestions in this book or drawing inferences from it.

The author and publisher specifically disclaim all responsibility for any liability, loss or risk, personal or otherwise, which is incurred as a consequence, directly or indirectly, from the use or application of any contents of this book.

Any and all product names referenced within this book are the trademarks of their respective owners. None of these owners have sponsored, authorized, endorsed, or approved this book.

Always read all information provided by the manufacturers' product labels before using their products. The author and publisher are not responsible for claims made by manufacturers.

This book was originally printed before 2014. This is an adapted reprint by Speedy Publishing LLC with newly updated content designed to help readers with much more accurate and timely information and data.

Speedy Publishing LLC

40 E Main Street, Newark, Delaware, 19711

Contact Us: 1-888-248-4521

Website: http://www.speedypublishing.co

REPRINTED Paperback Edition: ISBN: 9781635013221

Manufactured in the United States of America

Chapter 1 - Basic and Essentials of Health

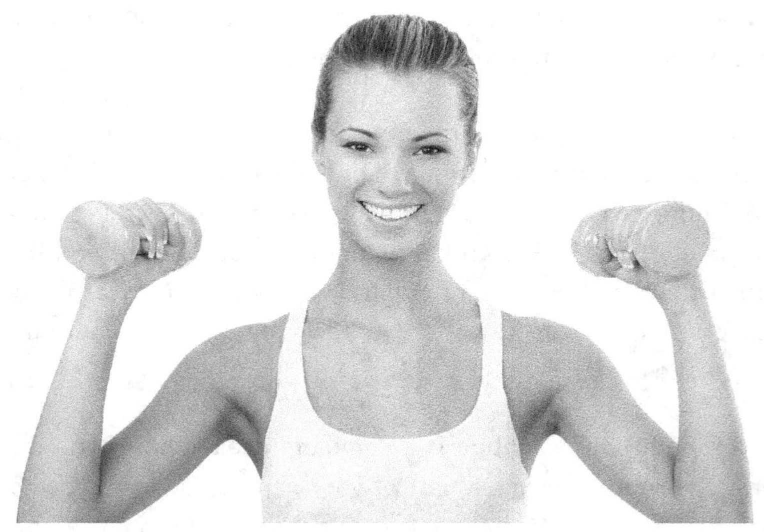

There is one common mistake which many people make when they decide to improve their bodies. This mistake is to not begin with adequate preparation. The first, and most essential, step in preparing to embark on a home workout program is to have a complete health clearance from your physician.

The most important reason for this is you may have a medical problem which you do not know exists. There are many health conditions which can worsen from strenuous exercise; there are some which can even be fatal. While you want to work toward that perfect body, you surely do not want to take unnecessary chances with your health or your life.

An evaluation from your physician will allow you to see if you have any extraordinary risk factors. This kind of check-up, which will take very little time or cost, is well worth the benefits. A clean bill of health will give you peace of mind-- and the go-ahead for your home workout.

The second reason is to find out whether you have any special limitations. For example, you may have had sprains or other types of injuries in the past. These can affect choosing the home workout that is right for you. Your doctor may advise you to modify certain kinds of exercise, or to avoid them altogether.

Visiting your physician before you begin a home workout regimen is necessary. If you have any health or medical problems, they need to be addressed before you start a home workout. Anything from a prior injury to an unknown heart condition can prevent you from getting the results you want from your workout. They can cause setbacks, and even disaster. A few minutes of your time beforehand can prevent all of this.

The best kind of evaluation is a complete evaluation. If you have not made routine exams a part of your general lifestyle, now is a good time to start. When you are serious about beginning a home workout regimen, you probably already know that it will affect your body. Whether you have exercised before or not, making a home workout a part of your everyday life will place stress and strain on your body. It will affect your muscles, your joints, your blood pressure, and every other part of your system. Your body will be working much harder than it ever did before, to move in the direction of your goals. This is why you need to know in advance that your body is ready for the task. It will help your workouts to proceed more smoothly, and without any unnecessary risks to your health.

A home workout is an exciting adventure. However, in addition to the effects it will have on your body, it will also affect your mind. From the increased blood flow which occurs during workouts, to the change in your blood-sugar levels, the physical benefits of exercise can affect your mood, spirits, and disposition. In order to ensure that these changes are positive and you gain as much from them as possible, you need to be prepared by knowing that you are healthy.

Many people have sustained permanent injuries, and worse, solely due to not being aware of medical problems or limiting conditions prior to starting a regimen of strenuous exercise. Others have become overwhelmed and discouraged, leading them to quit before seeing any positive results. Still others have given up, because they simply did not know what to expect from their new venture. In most cases, all of these repercussions can be avoided.

You want your new home workout routine to produce great results. You want the perfect body that you may have been dreaming of for many years. You want it all to come in the healthiest, safest, and most enjoyable manner, without any unnecessary risks or setbacks. Getting a complete evaluation from your doctor before you choose any exercise or purchase any equipment is the best way to make your home workout routine a positive experience.

When you know that you are healthy, and without any risk factors, you will have a double benefit. First, you can take on the workout routines of your choice without undue risk to your health; and second, you will have the peace of mind from knowing that your new venture is safe for you.

In the interest of your health and safety, make an appointment to see your doctor before you begin your new home workout. Not only is this the most sensible step, it will do wonders for your self-confidence. When you know that you are physically prepared for the home workout routines which you are about to begin, you can look forward to one of the best and most exciting experiences of your life.

Fitness is a Lifetime Investment

The time we put into our fitness at any time throughout our life is an investment in our future. Just as we try to build up our financial wealth, we should be doing the same with our health, as this will determine the quality of life as we age.

Consider the compound effect that smoking can have over the lifetime of a smoker and how detrimental it can be to their health. The opposite effect occurs when we do any form of fitness training even if it is only for a few minutes a day, or for short periods a few times a week.

We don't have to do hours of long intensive weight training 7 days a week to get fit.

To lose weight we don't need to go on strict diets that are too hard to maintain.

It takes a long time for most people to get fat and this usually occurs from eating just a little too much of the wrong foods too often.

If we are to reverse that situation and only reduce our calories by 100 per day, which is something that most people can achieve without too much difficulty, then the effect after a year or so can be quite dramatic.

If we were to walk for twenty minutes three or four times a week, we would be a lot healthier after a year of such exercise.

All these small changes won't encroach on our lifestyle to any extent but they can make the difference between normal activity when we age and the inability to get the most out of life.

The sooner we start to make these changes the more health we are investing in for our future. One of the best things about easy fitness like this is the fact that it gets even easier the more we do it.

Fitness is Often More about Attitude than Anything Else

It is our attitude that often determines our level of fitness. It is our attitude that will determine whether we want to sit on the couch or get out to the gym for a workout. The way we feel about our health and what we believe we have to give up in order to maintain it will be the deciding factor for our fitness.

If we believe that we have to miss out on some pleasures in life, such as watching the television or drinking with our friends then the price we have to pay for our fitness will seem too great.

Alternatively, if there are activities that we find can give us immediate satisfaction, and more satisfaction than long term good health, then often the choices we make will be determined by those activities rather than the ability to still be able to do those activities as we age.

It is not until it is too late that the wrong decisions, made because of our attitude towards health and fitness, determine the quality of life we are left with.

If only we could turn back the clock.

We need to look at our attitude towards health and ask ourselves the questions we would ask others if we were giving them advice.

Would you recommend someone starts smoking or drinking excessive alcohol if they were asking for advice on finding health for life? Not likely - Yet we make decisions like this every day that we will pay for dearly in the future.

Change your attitude and you can change your health, and in doing so you can expect to live life to the best of your ability. Exercise builds energy and energy is the source of all life. We have the opportunity to take this energy that is available, and all it takes to get our share is a positive attitude and action.

Chapter 2- Your Body and Its Needs

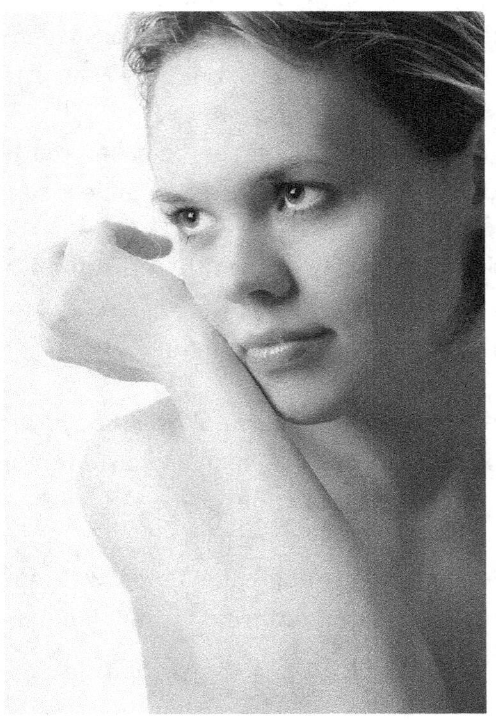

Good Nutrition

Nutrition is a study in itself and there is far more than could ever be covered in this course. There are however some nutrition basics that will help you to get better results from your training.

Many people are against taking supplements, but fitness training does place additional demands on our body and sometimes this can only be addressed by taking good supplements.

There are many different brands of supplements on the market and these have been developed due to the growth of the fitness industry and the fact that more people are concerned about their health.

Eating the right food will go a long way to supplying us with the nutrition that we need however even the best foods can't always supply us with the requirements of our busy lives.

One of the main food items (if it can be called that) that needs to be eliminated from our diets wherever possible is sugar.

Sugar will add nothing to your health and can do a whole lot of damage and cause problems such as diabetes to occur even for those people who are following good fitness training regimes.

You will need a level of quality complex carbohydrates to give you the energy to do your fitness training and also protein to help your muscles to recover and grow stronger.

These can be supplied through the foods we eat or by buying quality protein powders and nutritional supplements designed for people who train.

Recovery times can be shortened by supplements and taking supplements can enhance improvements in many aspects of fitness.

Good nutrition is probably the most important aspect of any fitness-training program, as it will ensure you are getting the maximum benefit from the work that you are putting in to your health. It can be quite costly but the rewards can be quite impressive too.

Nutrition Basics

Good nutrition is as important as the exercises we perform.

By eating wisely we are assisting our body to perform better in our chosen fitness program or sport.

The food we choose needs to be of high nutritional value to supply us with the necessary building blocks, in the form of vitamins and minerals to aid in recovery after strenuous workouts and to give us the energy to perform better during our exercise time.

Not only do we need to be supplying our body with the right vitamins and minerals but they also need to be in the correct balance.

When any one of these are out of balance and we are getting more or less than we should be, there will be an imbalance that will affect our progress.

This imbalance can even lead to illness, so buying good quality supplements is essential and knowing how much to take is also vitally important.

Another thing that needs to be addressed is your calorie intake as this will determine whether you are getting enough fuel to benefit your workouts or whether you are getting too much and adding fat to your body.

Foods high in refined sugar or animal fat should be avoided where possible, as they will be detrimental to your health.

If you are on a bodybuilding or resistance training program then you will need additional protein, as this is the muscle building food.

These foods, such as red meat will also supply you with the necessary B vitamins and Iron that are essential for strength training.

Other quality protein foods such as cheese, eggs, fish, poultry and milk should be included in your diet so you are getting variety in your diet.

These foods contain the essential amino acids, which are the building blocks of the body.

Vegetables are also another good source of amino acids however they generally have certain aminos missing and that is why the base protein foods listed above need to be included in your diet for complete nutrition.

A mix of foods is required as relying solely on meats for your protein can lead to other problems such as high levels of cholesterol.

Meat also is relatively high in fat, which is linked to the hardening of the arteries and heart disease. It is all about getting the correct balance with both your food and exercise.

Eating the Right Foods

Eating well is as important as the exercises you do each day.

It is not going to be very beneficial to your health if you have a diet of foods high in sugar and fat.

While the exercise will help you to achieve better health, the food you eat can do more harm than many people realize.

It is the fuel for your body and to eat the wrong food is like filling a petrol car with diesel.

You need energy to do your workouts and you need food to help your body to recover from those workouts.

Along with a fitness program it is wise to include good eating into your lifestyle.

This doesn't mean that you need to give up all the foods that you love to eat, but it does mean that you should be eating the correct foods most of the time.

We all have times when we feel like eating some fast foods or something that isn't high on the nutritional ladder but the basic foundation of our diet needs to be good food that can add to the quality of our health.

If most of your exercise is cardio work then you will need more carbohydrates to give you the energy to get through the workouts.

If on the other hand you are doing a lot of resistance training and trying to build muscle then you will eat more protein foods as these are the building blocks that help your muscles to build bigger and stronger after they have been broken down by strenuous weight training.

The food you eat before and after your exercise can have a huge effect on the benefits that you will get from your training. You can't expect to perform well at the gym if you have just finished a three-course meal, just as it would be difficult to go for a run after having too much to drink.

Doing so could actually endanger you where the body could become overloaded and stressed by having to deal with digestion and exercise.

Get a Better Sleep from Exercise

There's no doubt about the importance of regular and sound sleep for optimum health.

One of the benefits of regular exercise is the fact that it also helps to encourage better sleep patterns. By exercising there are benefits such as a reduction in stress levels that will also help you to relax more easily and this in turn will help you to sleep better.

You should not however exercise just before going to bed as the stimulation that you get from exercise can hinder your chance of going to sleep.

The best times to exercise are in the morning or early afternoon. This is not always convenient and many people are unable to exercise any time earlier than after work.

If this is the case then it is still best to exercise as early as possible and allow a little to unwind and relax before retiring for the night.

As your sleep patterns become more regular from the exercise your energy levels will increase from the additional sleep and this in turn will allow you to exercise more often and for longer periods.

With exercise and sleep complimenting one another you can make quite rapid gains in fitness and overall health provided you exercise consistently.

If you don't focus on getting good sleep, then there is a possibility you could wind up over training if you are exercising intensively.

Aside from good exercise and good sleep, you must always maintain good nutrition.

Nutrition also has a bearing on your ability to sleep well, so as you can see, you need balance in your life to get the most out of it.

When any element is missing and there is something out of balance all else suffers.

Even a little exercise will help a lot over a period of time, as will increasing your sleep and relaxation time.

The Importance of Water

With over 75% of our body made up of water there is no denying the need to remain hydrated at all times. If you are following a fitness program you will need to consume more water.

We are constantly losing water throughout the day and even at night while we sleep.

To remain hydrated we need to replace this water by drinking sufficient quantities so we never get thirsty.

With exercise we perspire more than normal and thereby lose more water, so anytime we exercise we need to drink more water than we would normally drink. If you feel thirsty then you are already getting dehydrated and your body is telling you to do something about it.

The problem with many people is their misunderstanding with what is suitable to drink.

There are so many flavored drinks available that people resort to these in preference to drinking water alone. Water doesn't have all the added sugars, preservatives and colorings that are detrimental to your health.

By remaining hydrated you will have more energy and this will allow you to perform better at the gym or your chosen exercise program.

It will also allow you to recover faster after a workout and reduce the chance of injury.

It is better to sip water constantly throughout the day, rather than try to meet your minimum requirements by drinking a lot all at one time. Most people live on a daily basis with less water than they should be having and that is why many people feel lethargic. If you are living in a hot climate you will need to consume more to compensate for the additional loss due to perspiration.

If you are consuming alcohol or caffeine you will need additional water to compensate for the diuretic effect that these have on the body. Have a glass of water before you go to bed at night and you should find you have increased energy when you wake up in the morning.

Also - You should have access to water when you are exercising and sip regularly from it.

This will help you to have a better workout and have more energy throughout your session.

CHAPTER 3- FITNESS ARMORY

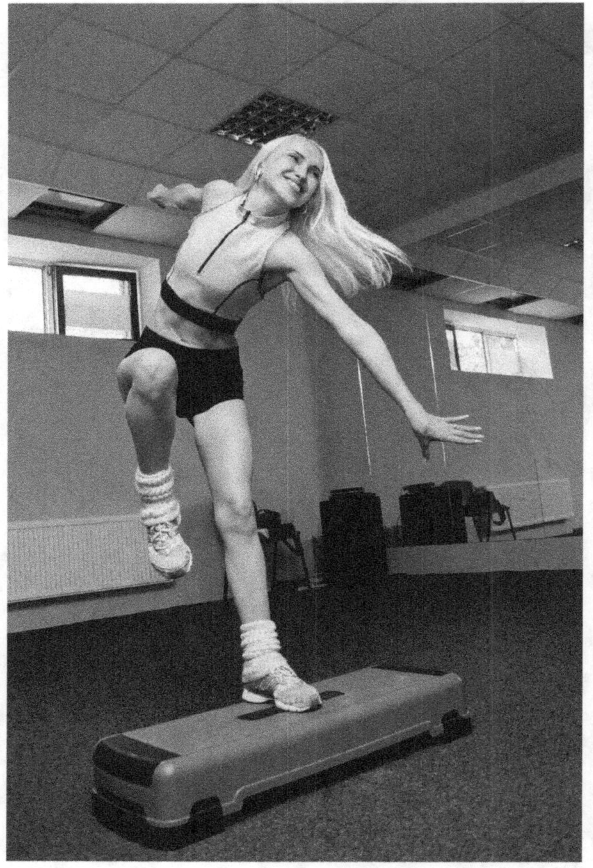

Fitness Apparel

Fitness apparel is far more than a fashion statement even if many people don't realize.

Good fitness apparel is designed specifically for the various sports or fitness training requirements to assist, protect and support the individual.

It might be designed to let the body breathe as in running vests or protect you from the weather.

It might be designed for support, with things like knee wraps aiding in heavy weight lifting exercises such as squats.

It might be designed to eliminate chafing as in cycling shorts or allow freedom of movement with yoga and Pilates gear.

It is important that you get the correct fitness apparel for the type of fitness training that you have chosen to pursue.

This will help you to perform better and will also reduce the chance of strains and injuries.

You should always choose apparel that is appropriate for the climate you will be exercising in, as an incorrect choice will hinder your performance.

The correct sizing and fit is also essential and you will often find that the better quality products are a lot more comfortable and perform better than the low cost items.

While you will need tighter fitting apparel for a sport such as cycling where wind resistance is an important factor, if your chosen fitness program is yoga you will be looking to buy loose fitting clothing that allows for ease of movement while performing your routines.

Once again the online sports stores often offer the best prices due to their reduced overheads and high sales volumes.

You do need to be careful when buying apparel online that you know your correct sizing although you can return goods that aren't suitable at most online stores.

The fashion element, while important to make you feel good, should be secondary to getting the correct fit, support and comfort that will ensure you perform better when training or competing.

Fitness Equipment

It is possible to get fit and improve your health with nothing more than a good pair of walking shoes.

Weather conditions and work commitments can make it difficult to find the time to do sufficient exercise to get the benefits that you are looking for.

Fortunately there is an answer, and that can be found in the vast array of home fitness equipment.

It is possible to buy a home gym for a reasonable price that can 'work' the whole body.

There are multi station gyms that offer as much benefits as a gym membership without the inconvenience of having to travel to the gym each time you want a workout.

Other benefits include, never having to wait for someone else to finish using the equipment, and not having to pay a membership fee year after year.

When these factors are taken into account it becomes clear how economical it is to invest in your own equipment.

By shopping online for fitness equipment there can be substantial savings due to the lower overheads of the online stores.

When searching for equipment you need to determine what your specific requirements are and then you can choose more wisely.

If you have no intentions of lifting heavy weights then a machine with a large weight stack will not get the use of the components you are paying for.

Everything from treadmills to heavy weight stacks are available to choose from and the range of equipment is matched by prices that can suit most budgets.

If the exercise equipment is in your house you are more likely to use it and having a sound system or television in the room can make your regime all the more enjoyable.

Whether it is the gym or a home gym we all have times when we don't feel inclined to exercise and those are the times when you won't want to be paying for a gym membership.

At least with your own equipment you can have a break for a period and it isn't going to cost you any more money.

Fitness Programs

To get the maximum benefit from your fitness training you should be following a specific program. You need to determine what you are trying to achieve with your fitness program and then design a course that will deliver the results you are after. If you have program to follow you will be able to record your progress and make changes as your level of fitness increases.

This is particularly important if you are doing resistance training, as it is difficult to know what changes to make if you don't know what your progress has been. Recording your progress will also spur you on to better performances. This helps your subconscious mind to drive you on as you realize the benefits of your training.

Record the number of repetitions that you achieve for each exercise and the weight that you use for each exercise and constantly challenge yourself to do better. Even increasing weights or repetitions in small increments can add up to some substantial improves in your levels of strength and fitness over time.

Without a record of progress many people tend to continue with the same weights or the same number of repetitions and wonder why they fail to achieve the levels that they hope for. If you are training to reshape your body it is also a good idea to record your starting point on film. Take a photo of yourself before you start your fitness program and at intervals along the way. It is best to only do this every few months as it can take time to see noticeable changes to your body. By recording this on film you can look back and the progress that you see visually and this will help to encourage and motivate you to continue with your program. There is nothing better than visual proof of accomplishment as a motivator.

Chapter 4- Getting Down, Sweaty and Dirty

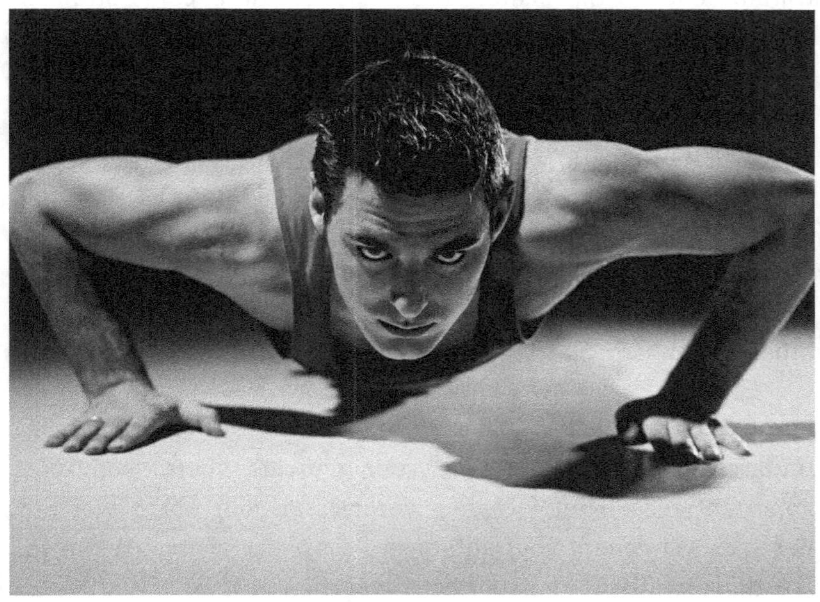

If you want that perfect body you have always dreamed of, you will need to exercise! The good news is that exercising does not have to mean boring routines which can soon become tiresome. There are three categories of exercises which will help you to gain that perfect body. When you have some information about each type, you can choose from amongst them to custom-design a home workout to meet your needs and personal preferences.

One form of exercise is known as pilates. While pilates have become increasingly popular during the last few years, it is not a modern concept at all. The basic principles of pilates go back as far as World War One, when they were developed in Germany by Joseph Pilate.

These exercise routines are great for the overall body, while placing much emphasis on the areas which most people find to be troublespots. Whether you are hoping to lose unwanted fat, or develop as much healthy muscle as possible, pilates are an excellent choice for your home workout routine. Your abs, hips, buttocks, and thighs will all benefit from pilates. Your muscles will become stronger, more flexible, and healthier.

There are many different exercise routines in the pilates category. Some of the most popular are "the Hundred" and "the Roll-Up," which will do wonders for your abdominal muscles; and "the Single-Leg Stretch" and "the Double-Leg Stretch," which will tone your buttocks and hips as well as your abdominal region. Many of the pilates exercises do not require any kind of exercise equipment other than a basic mat.

Aerobics is another popular form of exercise. While aerobics routines will assist in toning your muscles, there is a more important reason for including aerobics in your home workout. Aerobics will benefit your entire cardiovascular system. When you are thinking about that perfect body, health is as important as appearance. Adding aerobics exercise to your workout routine will strengthen your heart and your lungs. It will promote better health, as well as making your workout a truly exhilarating experience.

Calisthenics may already be familiar to you. You may remember some calisthenics exercises from your school days. However, you may not have known how beneficial they can be in helping you to create the body of your dreams. Whether or not you enjoyed calisthenics as a youngster, they will go a long way in sculpting that perfect body.

There are many different calisthenics exercises from which to choose, so you can easily incorporate some of your favorites into your home workout. Some of the most common calisthenics exercises are jumping jacks, abdominal crunches, push-ups, sit-ups, and squats. They will get your blood pumping, and tone and firm your body. It will be fun to see how exercises you learned as a child can be so useful in helping you to create the perfect body you want today.

When you have custom-designed the exercise routines you wish to include in your home workout, you are partway to developing the workout which you will do each session. However, there are a couple of other points to consider before your workout regimen is complete. These extra points will make your workouts less stressful on your body.

First, regardless of the types of exercises you have chosen, you must begin each session with a warm-up. A brief period of basic stretching and bending will give your body the preparation it needs to be ready for a workout. This little preliminary can make quite a difference. When your body is readied beforehand, the exercising will flow more naturally and smoothly.

Second, a cooling-down period should be at the end of every home workout. The same kinds of stretching and bending motions that you used to warm up will help your body to conclude the workout. It will prepare your body for rest.

It is not difficult to choose the forms of exercise that are best for you. You can start by thinking about the types of exercise you like the most, and conform them to your specific needs. You can tone the areas which are most in need of attention, or aim for an overall workout which will benefit your entire body.

It is important to choose exercises which you will not tire of, so that you will be motivated to do your workout on a regular basis. If you keep your expectations reasonable, and demonstrate self-discipline, you will be pleased with the results. You can begin to see your body's shape and strength improve within a relatively short period of time. The perfect body you have always wanted can be yours-- and it all starts with custom-designing your own exercise routine.

When to Use Weights

When you think of gaining that perfect body, thoughts of weights may come to mind. Whether this is positive or negative depends on your opinion. While planning a great home workout can include the use of weights, a workout can be done without them. In addition, there are a number of different kinds of weights, if you do decide to use them.

One form of weights are known as dumbbells. These are good to use when doing exercises while standing. While dumbbells can greatly tone the muscles in your arms, shoulders, and upper torso, they can also assist in toning your abdominal muscles.

Dumbbells can be found in a variety of different weights. When you are beginning your workouts, it is a good idea to start with lighter dumbbell, and increase the weight as your body becomes accustomed to the workouts.

A second form of weights is barbells. They are generally used while lying flat. While the power exercise known as bench-pressing is popular amongst professional body-builders and other athletes, you can easily make it a part of your own home workout routine. As bench-pressing places a considerable amount of strain on the body, especially the abdomen, it is essential to choose light weights when you are beginning your workout routines. Otherwise, this strain could cause permanent damage to your muscles. When you choose lighter weights, you can easily work up to heavier weights as your body becomes accustomed to this practice.

While dumbbells and barbells are available in various weights, there is an additional feature which can be useful to you. Dumbbells and barbells are both available in a solid, one-piece style, and in a style which allows you to take off and add on weights as your needs change. The latter can be the most beneficial to your workout routine, as you can continue to adjust the amount of weight you use to reflect the progress you make in your workouts.

You may also be wondering if you can get that perfect body without using any weights at all. The answer to this is yes, it is possible, but it is likely to take longer. The exercises you do with weights direct the focus to specific points in your body. The use of the weights helps these points to tone and strengthen quicker and easier. Power exercises done with weights will give you that perfect body faster, but this does not mean you cannot get the body you want without using them. If you are prepared to work harder and longer, you can reach your goal without using weights.

If you have decided that weights are a good addition to your home workout, there are some safety tips to make your workout better, more pleasurable, and without undue risk. Please do not simply order weights and begin using them without considering these tips first.

One tip is to be sure you choose the right weights. If you are not accustomed to using this kind of workout equipment, it cannot be stressed too strongly that you should select light weights. Whether you are considering barbells, dumbbells, or both, you do not want to put too much strain on your body and risk injury.

Another tip is to ensure your safety when you work out with weights. While this is true for exercising in general, maneuvering weights in a standing position means wearing appropriate workout gear. You should have sneakers or similar shoes with non-slip rubber soles. You should also avoid wearing clothes that are too loose or long sleeves.

It is also important to be sure that you are working out on a safe floor. Slipping or falling can be especially dangerous if you are working out with weights. You should avoid floors with rugs, carpeting, tile, and other potentially hazardous material or coverings. Whether you create your own home gym, or simply devote one particular part of your home to a workout space, you must keep your safety in mind when you work out with your weights.

Working out with weights can give you that perfect body! It will also invigorate your entire system. Your heart and lungs will greatly benefit when you make working out with weights a part of your home workout routine. If you keep all of these tips in mind, start slowly, and do not demand overnight results, you will be amazed at how quickly you do begin to see results.

Your body will not only feel stronger, it will actually be stronger. The new tone you will see in your muscles will be beyond compare. That perfect body you have always dreamed of will be more than just a dream-- it will start to take shape, and be in the best condition of your life.

Chapter 5- Machine and Weights Handling

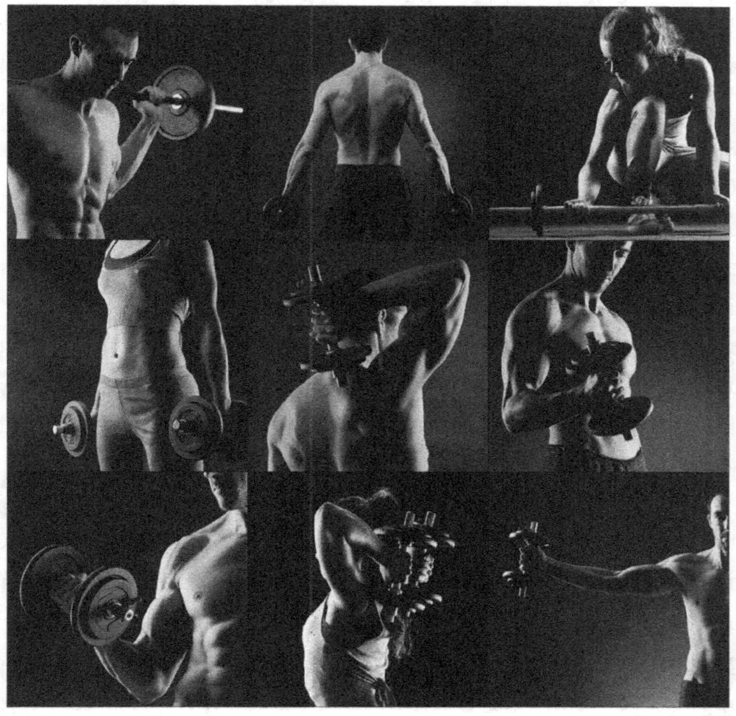

One mistake many people make when preparing to do home workouts is to go overboard in purchasing exercise equipment. They end up wasting money on expensive equipment they do not really need, and cluttering their homes with products they will not use. When you are preparing to do home workouts, some tips will help you to decide what kinds of equipment are suitable for you.

One point to consider is the amount of space you have in the area where you plan to work out. A good rule of thumb is that you probably do not need more equipment than you can comfortably fit in that space. Even the smallest workout space can accommodate your exercise equipment if you do not purchase unnecessary products.

A second factor is cost. While you may be tempted to purchase all of the popular equipment you have seen advertised, the expense is rarely worth it. You do not have to equip your workout space to rival a gymnasium-- you can have that great body without it.

The third factor is your goal. As you probably already know what you hope to accomplish from your home workouts, selecting the right equipment will help you to reach your goal.

You should also consider your own preferences. If you are like most people, there are certain things which you like and certain things which you dislike. Even if you think specific types of exercise equipment are absolutely necessary, they will not get much use if you hate to use them. When you focus on your preferences, you will be more likely to get the exercise equipment that is best suited to you.

While taking these factors into consideration can assist you in choosing the right exercise equipment, there are a few types of equipment which are especially beneficial to the person who is beginning a new home workout regimen. With a little comparison-shopping, you can find them at a relatively low price to fit your budget. It is not necessary to buy name brands, or the most expensive model on the market. You can be price-conscious, while giving your new home workout the boost it needs to be successful and fun!

One piece of exercise equipment that is easy to use, enjoyable, and beneficial, is a stationary bike. A stationary bike can be the ideal way to warm up before your regular workout, or a nice change as a mini-workout in itself. A good stationary bike is adjustable, so that it will feel custom-fit for your personal comfort. It will provide all of the benefits of riding a bicycle-- right in your own home. It is a great way to exercise in general, as well as to focus on those troublesome spots. If you use a stationary bike on a regular basis, it will help to firm your hips, buttocks, and thighs. This is one type of exercise equipment that will make working out feel like play.

A treadmill will also provide special benefits. If you are new to working out, using a treadmill can help to increase your physical endurance. You will become able to breathe better, and gain better strength in your heart and lungs. As a perfect body has as much to do with increasing your health to its very best as it does with your appearance, a treadmill should be on your must-have list of home exercise equipment.

A rowing machine is another popular piece of exercise equipment. When your goal is that perfect body, you will be delighted with how quickly the regular use of a rowing machine begins to tone your abdominal muscles, your arms, and your shoulders. Not only will a rowing machine help to strengthen your upper body, it will increase your body's firmness. Your upper body will start to take on a better shape as your muscles become more well-defined.

If you have a large area of your home to devote to your workouts, and plenty of money to spare, you can choose a number of other types of exercise equipment for your workouts. However, you can have the best possible start to that perfect body without spending a lot of money or using a lot of space. When you begin your new home workouts with only these three pieces of exercise equipment, you may soon decide that you do not really need any others.

In addition, considering basic home exercise equipment as a worthwhile investment is a positive way to look at it. When you purchase these products, you are not only taking the first step toward creating the body of your dreams, you are also making strides toward a healthier body that can last for a lifetime. Even if you have only a small amount of money to put into your home workouts, these few pieces of exercise equipment will be well worth the investment. They will help you to reach your goal of a great-looking body, while increasing your overall health at the same time.

Machines and Weights

Using a combination of weights and machines for training will give you the best of both worlds, with the ability of machines allowing you to use more weight under a controlled environment, and the free weights helping to stimulate the synergistic muscles for balance and control.

Add to this some cardio work for aerobic fitness and you are getting all that anyone could hope for in a fitness program. These types of programs can be developed for the gym, and with the abundance of good home gym equipment, they can also be used at home.

Many times you can get a better workout from home as you won't need to wait on other people to finish their exercises before you can use the equipment.

Machines also allow you to use heavy weights in complete safety where you will need to be a little more cautious with free weights if you don't have someone to assist with your training.

Age can determine which one would be best to use. The safety factor is very important for children and elderly people.

There are many types of machines available and they all have their benefits over one another. There are machines that have weight stacks, which can be quite heavy, and then there are machines that use cables and rods to offer resistance.

Some are portable and able to be moved and folded away whereas some of the big weight stack machines are too heavy to move easily. These are factors that need to be considered when buying machines whereas free weights can be used almost anywhere, from inside the house to the back yard.

With free weights you will need to consider a weight bench to ensure you can perform sufficient exercises to build most muscles of your body. There is no real maintenance required with free weights, as they will still perform well even if you were to leave them to rust.

Chapter 6- Novelty Exercise That Do Work

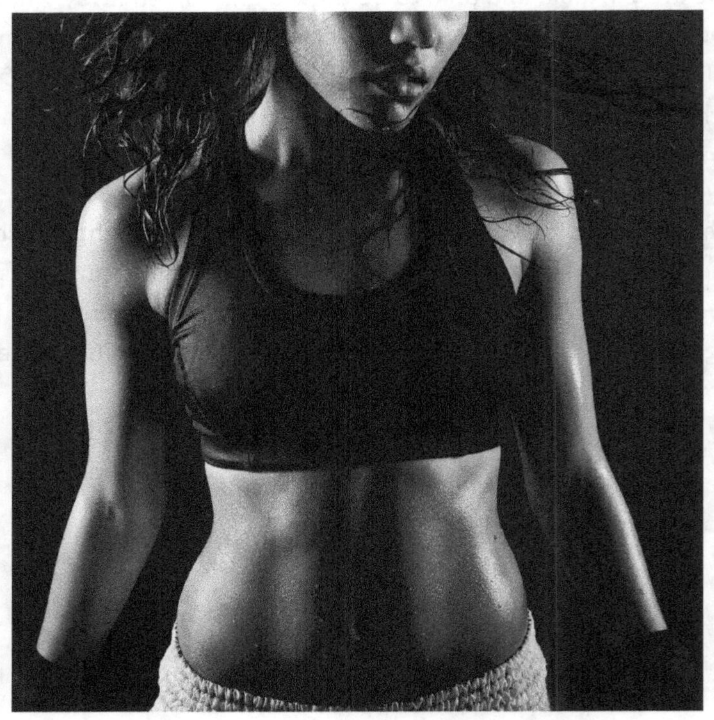

You may be well-motivated and looking forward to beginning your new home workout regimen. At the same time, you may be wondering if you could benefit from something more. You may be unsure of whether you are completely prepared to do it all on your own. If you think that you need a little extra help, it could very well put you on the right track.

Fitness Gimmicks

There are many different fitness items advertised on the television every day of the week.

Some of these are actually very good for helping gain and maintain a strong healthy body but there are others that can best be described as gimmicks. If anything promises to give you the body of a bodybuilder or fitness model overnight then it is something that you should steer clear of. It is not possible to make drastic changes over night and promises to that effect are untrue.

You cannot lose vast amounts of weight in a few days or reduce your waist measurements dramatically overnight even if you were to starve for a few days. This is all advertising hype to get you to part with your money. Unfortunately this type of advertising can often make people skeptical about the benefits of other quality pieces of fitness equipment.

Progress should always be gradual whether it is for weight loss or weight and muscle gain. Nothing good happens overnight and there is some effort required to get results.

People promoting gimmick products are trying to sell a dream. You can't expect rock hard abs in an instant if you have been over weight for the last twenty years. You can however, expect to get good results from using quality fitness equipment on a regular basis that has been designed correctly to target specific areas of the body.

If you are constantly looking for a fast fix all you will get is a delayed start to a quality fitness program that could deliver the results you long for. When you see the results that can be achieved with something as simple as a barbell and free weights you will understand that fitness is not about the equipment you have but the actions you take to improve your health.

Circuit Training is Fun

Circuit training is a fun way to get fit. It is also an excellent form of training to help people to stay motivated as you get a variety of exercises to perform in the course of a training session.

A well-designed fitness-training program will also target all the muscles of the body so you will be getting a full body workout at each session.

Combined with upbeat music that many gyms have on with circuit training, the time tends to pass a lot faster and the fun aspect ensures people are happy to return to the gym and that can only be good for their health.

If you are not a member of a gym it is possible to design your own circuit-training program for home.

The equipment you have will determine much of the program but it is possible to design a circuit-training program based around exercises that only use your own body weight.

It can also include indoor or outdoor activity and include walking and running as part of the training program. A stereo at home or an iPod for outside training can add to the fun just as you would get as a member of a gym.

You can design the program to target any areas of your body that you desire and it can be fun creating your own training program and making changes to your training as you progress.

As will all forms of training it is good to keep a record of your results and always challenge yourself to do better. Carrying a note book and pen might seem like a bit of a hassle but the record of your progress can be inspiring and there will be sufficient time in between the exercises to jot down these notes.

It can be quite surprising sometimes how we forget how much we have progressed over the course of a few weeks or months.

Yoga for Fitness

Realizing the benefits of yoga can add a whole new dimension to your levels of fitness and flexibility. There was a time when many people considered yoga to be the exercise that elderly people and housewives would do during the day.

This couldn't be further from the truth and some yoga routines can deliver a more strenuous workout than many professional sportsmen and women can endure. In fact, the recent rise in popularity of yoga has been helped by the many professional sports people, who have adopted this as part of their fitness training, to assist with flexibility and help reduce injuries.

Yoga can be tailored to suit anybody's requirements from the very elderly to the professional sports person.

By stretching the muscles in controlled poses the flexibility that can be garnered will reduce the chance of torn or strained muscles on the playing field.

With the amount of money that is invested in professional sports now there is a need to ensure that the sports person is fit and able to perform throughout the season.

Time out due to injury is too expensive to ignore and that is why yoga is becoming more popular.

Yoga is a low impact form of exercise and as such can be used under guidance even when people are suffering from injuries and it can also assist in the recovery process.

It is also excellent for stress reduction. Apart from the positive aspects of increased flexibility, stress reduction and improved mobility, yoga is also very good for improving strength. Standing poses where a position is held for a length of time can improve leg strength and at the same time improve the yoga student's balance. There are so many areas of fitness that yoga encompasses that it is one of the best all-round body and mind workouts that you could do.

Pilates for Fitness

Like Yoga there has been a vast increase in the number of people who are using Pilates as their preferred form of fitness.

Once again it is the professional sports people who have helped popularize Pilates recently as they strive for a more rounded training regime that will help to reduce injury, add strength and flexibility and assist in their recovery if they are unfortunate enough to get injured.

Pilates focuses on the core postural muscles, which are the abdominals, lower back muscles, the hips and buttocks.

By building a strong core structure this strength can flow out to all the other muscles of the body from this center.

Pilates requires concentration where the muscles are controlled throughout all movements, which help to build strength. There have since been some variations on the base method taught in

Pilates by the original founder Joseph Pilates, but they are all centered on this same principal of core training.

This is especially useful for athletes in many sports and it is a popular method of fitness training for people of all ages.

By teaching this control with fluid movements Pilates offers a complete body workout and in doing so can help to reduce the incidence of injury that can occur when participating in other sports activities.

There are machines that are used for a lot of the Pilates exercises and these can be quite expensive. Throughout the country there are dedicated Pilates gyms that have the correct equipment and instructors to ensure that the movements are being performed correctly.

Learning the Pilates techniques correctly is essential as these movements if performed incorrectly could do more harm than good. There are also various videos and DVD's available that will teach you the Pilates techniques if you prefer to do your exercises at home. It is a good alternative for people who like something a little different than yoga.

One possibility is to enlist the aid of a personal trainer. It is not necessary to have a personal trainer at your side for the duration of your workouts-- some input when you are starting out can be very beneficial.

A personal trainer can help to customize your home workout regimen, if you are uncertain of what is right for you. He can also advise you of what to expect from your workouts. If you do not know how to deal with discomfort in your muscles, or how long you can reasonably expect to wait before you see results, a personal fitness trainer can answer all of your questions.

A second possibility is a short-term membership at a gym. Even if you plan to do your workouts in your own home, there is much to be gained from a few visits to a gym. You can see workout equipment in use, which can help you to decide which types of equipment you want for your home. You can interact with others who are working out, which will help you to see what you yourself need to do, and the results which you can expect. You can take this entire knowledge home with you, to put to use in your own workouts.

Another possible extra is for your home workouts to utilize the buddy system. While some people do very well at any venture on their own, others do much better if they are in the company of likeminded friends, or even family members. If you are in the latter category, encouraging others to join you in your home workouts can be useful to both you and the others in your life. Mutual support can be quite motivating. Even healthy, good-spirited competition can make your workouts more enjoyable and more oriented toward results.

The buddy system is not for everyone. There are many who do much better with working out alone. You probably already know which category describes you the best. Whichever one you choose, it should be the method that works for you.

An additional factor is your own level of motivation. There are many people who want great results, but are not sure that they have what it takes to get there. You may wonder if you will always have the time to devote to your workouts, or if you might become tired or discouraged and tempted to quit, or whether you may decide that it really is not worth the effort. If you want your home workout routine to be a success, and to give you that perfect body, it is a good idea to address these concerns in advance.

Everyone becomes discouraged at times, and no one is one-hundred-percent motivated each and every day. For your workouts to be a success, without the worry of quitting before you reach your goal, you should have a plan for how to deal with those less-than-ideal days before they occur.

As each person has his own method of getting things done, consider the method that works for you. How do you prime yourself to do something when you really do not feel like doing it? It could be a task at work, a household chore, or even something you usually like. No one is at his best every single day, but this does not mean you can afford to neglect whatever you must do. This includes your home workout routines.

When you know the method you use in your everyday life, you can apply the same methods to your workouts. Perhaps it involves getting yourself in a certain frame of mind. Perhaps you might give yourself a small treat, chat with a friend, or promise yourself a reward for a job well done. Whatever works for you, to help you to be motivated when you do not feel motivated at all, can be a wonderful aid to keeping you on track. If you have such a plan in advance, you will be less likely to skip your workouts, and more enthusiastic about doing them.

You may decide that you do not need any of these little "extras" at all. You may be the type of person who can commit a specific period of time into your daily schedule for workouts, and stick to it on a regular basis, without fail. If this sounds accurate, good for you! However, giving yourself the option for extra help when you need it is not a sign of weakness. It only means that you know yourself well enough to be aware that you may require a bit of extra help to be consistent with your home workouts. If it will help you to stay on the right track, incorporating some extra help into your basic workout plan is a positive step. It can keep you on the track toward success!

Chapter 7- Consistency is the Key

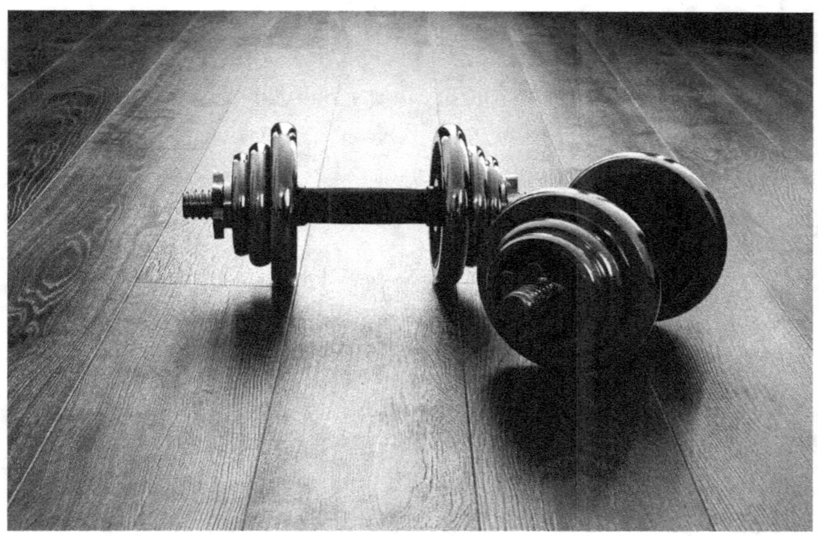

The Benefits of Fitness

There are many benefits from regular fitness training that will have ongoing positive effects on the quality of your life.

Prevention of illness is one of the most important aspects of maintaining a healthy body.

It has been proven that regular exercise and the heightened levels of health that develops from this exercise can help to reduce the incidence of diseases such as diabetes, heart diseases and strokes.

Exercise can reduce hypertension and many other ailments.

As well as this, fitness training can help people have a more positive outlook on life and improve their self-confidence.

Regular exercise releases endorphins in the body that help to fight the symptoms of depression and give us a feeling of happiness.

It only takes a little more than 10 minutes of continuous exercise for the body to start releasing endorphins.

Another chemical that is increased in the body during and after exercise is serotonin. This occurs in the central nervous system and is also responsible for making us feel happier and reducing the possibility of depression.

Serotonin also assists in getting better sleep and that in turn helps with better workouts through increased energy.

Fitness can become addictive as we start to realize these benefits of feeling better in both the mind and the body.

The more fitness training we do the more of these 'positive' chemicals are released into our body and we get happier and healthier with each passing day.

By reshaping our body with exercise, and particularly resistance training, we feel better about ourselves and this also helps to build self-esteem and self-confidence.

This flows over into all aspects of life and we begin to find that even work and family life benefit from the more positive energy that fitness training brings.

Regular exercise is the key to success as energy builds with consistency and this make the training easier to handle and more enjoyable.

Fitness Plateaus

We will all hit plateaus in our training progress whether we are beginners or advanced fitness experts.

Even the top bodybuilders, and those who are taking steroids will plateau from time to time and it is something that we need to understand to breakthrough.

The first thing many people will do is to increase their training intensity.

This is the wrong move for most beginners and intermediate people as it quickly leads to over training.

Many times these plateaus will come about when the body is crying out for a bit more time to recover and rebuild.

Inexperienced fitness enthusiasts will see this as a sign that they need to push harder to continue their development and so begins an ever more difficult time where the training intensity increases but the results diminish.

If this problem isn't addressed soon enough it can lead to illness as the immune system gets overloaded with the loads that are being placed upon it.

If you find that you aren't making progress with your training then it might be time to reduce your training intensity, either by lifting lighter weights, working out for a shorter time, or in the case of aerobic exercises like running, reduce the distances and times of your training for a week or two.

In some cases where the training has been particularly intense you might even need to take a few days or a week off where you have a complete break and come back rejuvenated. The more you exercise the better you get at reading your body and understanding when it is time to train harder and when it is time to take a break.

You might also need to consider having a backup training plan for these times where you will do something completely different to maintain fitness but still have a rest from your usual regime. If you usually run for fitness you might try swimming for a week or two before coming back to your running training again.

Fitness Should be Fun

Gaining and maintaining your fitness can be fun and should be fun.

Anything that is seen as a chore is something that most people will try to avoid and it will make it difficult to maintain for any period of time.

Unlike a job where we get paid for doing something that we might not always enjoy, the rewards from fitness are something that are difficult to place a value on.

Obviously the value of good health is more important that most things in life but it is so easy to discount, that we need to look at the fitness program that we will be using to ensure it will be fun and we will continue to use it.

There are so many different ways of keeping fit and many of these can be as enjoyable as a walk in the park with your dog or a swim in the pool every day.

If you are starting on a fitness program that you find difficult and unappealing from day one then there is a good possibility that you will not follow through and get the benefits that you expect from the program

You would be better off choosing a program that might not deliver the same results in the same time but one that you know you will follow through until the end. If you can find some form of fitness training that you really enjoy doing then you can make it a lifetime activity and enjoy improved health for as long as possible.

Your fitness program should be something that you look forward to when you wake each day. The fitter you get, and the more benefits that you see from your fitness the more likely you are going to enjoy what you are doing. Your perspective of training will change, as you get fitter, so you might find that you need to reassess the program you are on and change it as your fitness level increases.

Chapter 8- Women and Their Exercise Needs

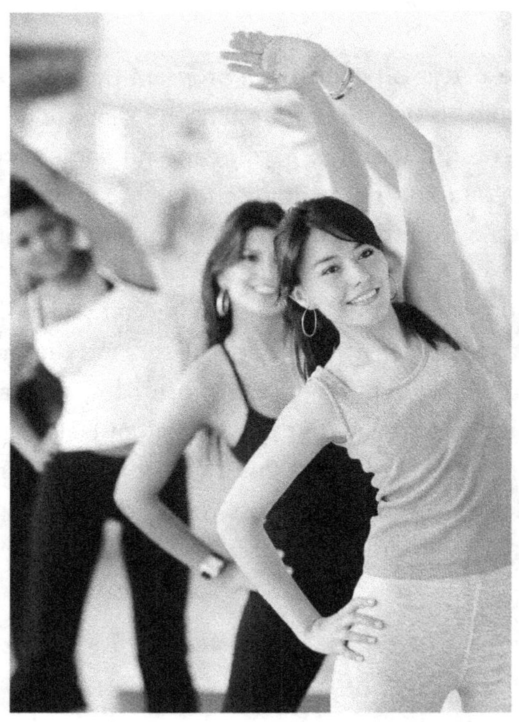

These days, home workouts are as popular amongst women as they are for men. Women have a natural desire to look and feel their best, too. This is evident by the large number of women who join gyms, purchase exercise equipment, and try various diets. While being more physically attractive and healthier are sensible goals for women, women who wish to begin home workouts do have special circumstances.

One topic is working out during pregnancy. You may have heard "old wives' tales" who claim that no exercise at all is safe when you are pregnant, and you may also heard that virtually nothing is off limits. If you are pregnant, or planning to become pregnant, you may be unsure of which point of view to believe.

With your doctor's approval, working out during pregnancy can be very beneficial. In fact, starting a home workout routine prior to becoming pregnant can prepare your body for this exciting adventure. The better shape your body is in, the easier and more comfortable your pregnancy and childbirth will be for you. It will also make returning to your pre-pregnant state easier and faster after your baby is born.

However, you should be sensible about your home workouts. Your goal is to get your body in its ideal condition, not to overtax your strength or put unreasonable demands on your body. The home workout routine you choose should reflect making your body stronger and more limber, and improving your muscle tone. It is unwise to go to extremes with working out while you are pregnant. If you really want to lift weights, it is best to wait until after your baby is born!

A second topic involves the female anatomy in general. Even when pregnancy is not an issue, you must still take this into consideration. Although it should be obvious, your body is made differently than that of your husband or brother. First, workout routines which place an extreme degree of stress on the abdominal and pelvic regions can indeed cause damage to the internal organs. This is something to keep in mind when you are choosing your home workout program.

In addition, the female muscles are not as prepared for strenuous routines as those of a man's. This does not mean that you cannot obtain the perfect body you want. It does mean taking on less, especially at the beginning, and proceeding slower. If working out is new to you, it is not a good idea to risk tearing muscles by attempting to do too much, too soon.

Health and Fitness Buff

Whether your body is petite or full-figured, athletic or out of shape, you can have the perfect body of your dreams. In order to avoid the risk of unnecessary injuries, common sense is the key. After all, the purpose of working out is to get your body in its best possible shape, not to incur damage which can slow you down or even become permanent.

The woman who does not have pregnancy as a factor should assess her personal situation before planning a home workout routine. The current condition of your body, and how familiar it is with exercise in general, are two points to consider. If you are already athletic, and used to a moderate amount of exercise on a regular basis, you have more leeway than the woman who has never exercised and is quite out of shape.

Thinking about your goals is a positive way to begin. Do you want to increase your overall health, stamina, and be your most attractive? Firming and toning your body can give you a glowing, youthful appearance, regardless of your age. The body that is strong and fit is also a healthier body. It will reduce your risk of developing many kinds of illnesses and diseases, make everyday life a joy, and can even add years to your lifespan. There is much more to a great body than simply looking good in a swimsuit!

Your goals should be sensible. While you may be able to obtain the body of a female bodybuilder, this is not a common goal for most women. You probably want to get the body you have in its best possible condition, so that you will feel and be more attractive. You probably also want the strong, toned body that reflects good health.

If these are your goals, physical fitness is your answer. You can choose the home workout routines which not only move you toward your goal, but are also much fun to do. Your home workout program will be much more satisfying, and you will be more likely to reach your goals, if you do not start with routines that are too physically-taxing or dull.

Starting with simple routines instead will give you two benefits. First, you will be less likely to incur injury; and second, when you choose fun routines, you will be more likely to continue them faithfully. Your workouts will be something to look forward to, each and every day.

Any woman can have a more attractive, healthier body. Most women can obtain amazing results. The key is to take your circumstances into consideration, and begin your workouts with enthusiasm. You can have that perfect body you have always wanted if you start slowly and proceed with consistency.

Personalized Fitness Programs

Whether you are using resistance training, yoga, pilates, aerobic fitness training or one of the many methods to get fit and lead a healthier life there is one important ingredient that you must have and that is a personalized fitness program.

No two people have the same requirements to reach their optimum health and this has to be represented in the choice of fitness program and even within that choice of the specific actions that are necessary.

By this I mean that, if for instance you choose resistance training for your fitness program, you will need a personalized program of exercises that will suit your body type, the condition of your health, your time restraints and so forth.

The same will apply to a yoga program. While you might join a yoga class for your preferred form of exercise, you will need to place more emphasis on those exercises that will assist the areas of your body that need help the most.

The reason for this need to have a personalized program is simply because you will want to get the best results in the shortest time to get to a good level of health and fitness without losing motivation.

There is nothing less motivating than a lack of progress and that is precisely what will happen if you don't have a fitness program that addresses all your needs. There are programs that will serve as the basis for the majority of people but they will need to be adjusted and modified to personal requirements.

Keeping a fitness diary will help as it will show which areas are progressing well and where changes will need to be made to get more improvement.

The information from the data that you record will be the source of your fast track to health and fitness.

Chapter 9- Now is the Time To Get in Shape!

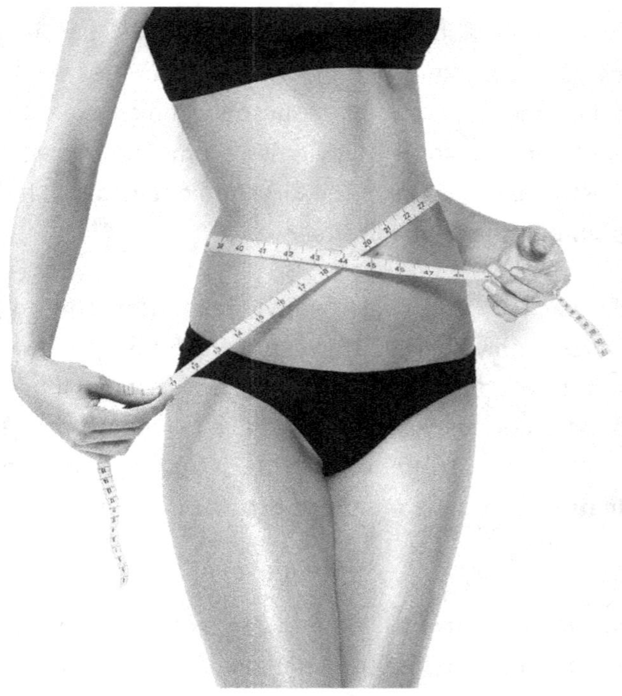

You are thinking about that perfect body. You may wonder if you have what it takes to obtain it. You may have a special situation which is leading you to doubt whether a home workout is for you. After all, the idea of starting a workout routine, and aiming for the body of your dreams, is quite new to you.

The good news is that home workouts are a great option for nearly anyone. Even if there is something different about your particular situation, you can turn it into something positive for working out.

One situation is the person who has neglected his body for many years. Not only has he become out-of-shape, flabby, and weak, the body that is not properly cared for often suffers in terms of health.

You may be considerably overweight, even obese. If this sounds like you, you may be thinking that a home workout program would be useless, if not hazardous.

In this kind of situation, slowly-but-surely is the key to success. Beginning your workout program with easy exercises will help your body to become accustomed to its new adventure. While it is necessary to follow your physician's recommendations, it is not impossible for you to move in the direction of a healthy, fit body. In fact, it is simpler than you may believe.

The body that has been neglected will take more time to get into shape. This is only logical. However, you must not give up on yourself before you begin! You may be carrying more than a hundred extra pounds, and you may have fallen into the sedentary lifestyle of a couch-potato. With effort, hard work and determination, you can shed those extra pounds, and be physically fit and healthy again!

A second situation involves youngsters who are longing for that perfect body. It must be stressed that children and adolescents who are still growing should not take on a strenuous workout routine without their doctor's approval. This does not mean that working out is not suitable for children and teens. It only means that special attention must be focused on their growth stage.

When you keep this in mind, developing a good home workout program is one of the best things you can do for your child. He will learn to associate exercise with fun, and he will become stronger and healthier at the same time. When you provide your youngster with a workout program that is appropriate for his age and stage of physical development, you are teaching him good habits that will benefit him throughout his entire lifetime.

Many people who have physical impairments or disabilities also want to improve their bodies. It can give them more self-confidence, and be a boost to their overall health. If you have a disability or a medical condition which could interfere with the safety of a home workout program, it is advisable to check with your doctor before you begin. He can help you to customize a workout that is based on your special needs.

Some people have the idea that working out is only for young adults. They may believe that once a person reaches a certain age, working out is useless, and even dangerous. The good news is that nearly anyone who is reasonably healthy is not only capable of working out, but can benefit from a solid workout program.

You may be forty or sixty years of age, and not at all pleased with the condition of your body. You may be listening to friends or family members who tell you that you must accept this as a natural part of aging. This is not true at all! While your age may require you to impose sensible limitations on working out, you will be delighted with the results. You can have the fit, firm body that you recall from decades in the past, increase your overall health, and have a general sense of wellbeing. Working out at home can be the best decision you have ever made!

Almost anyone can benefit from working out. Most people can gain positive results. If you have any of these or other special situations, do not dismiss the idea of a home workout program. Regardless of your situation, a program can be custom-tailored, just for you. Your doctor and a physical fitness trainer can provide the advice you need to get on the right track.

As long as you proceed in a sensible manner, and keep your expectations reasonable, the odds are on your side that you will be successful. Home workouts are not only for the young, the person with unlimited time and resources, or the person who has athletics in mind. The benefits you gain from your workouts will have you convinced within a very short period of time. Anyone can look his best, and feel his best-- and this means you, regardless of your personal situation.

About the Author

Steve Mallari is a fitness guru based in California. He is currently working as a fitness consultant for the top makers of exercise equipment. As a vegan, he pushes for sustainable living and organic farming. He is famous for using plant alternatives to animal produce as a means to increase muscle. Steve has appeared in several podcasts to talk about his suggested best practices in the area of health and fitness.

This book was designed to assist those who want to turn their health around for the better as well as keep the reader abreast with new techniques can fast-track you to proper fitness. Steve's very much sought after professional advice is compiled in this best-seller book.